Beautiful Nails

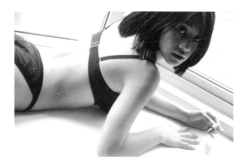

Written by Emma Ranson

KUDOS

Published by Kudos, an imprint of Top That! Publishing plc.
Copyright © 2005 Top That! Publishing plc,
Tide Mill Way, Woodbridge, Suffolk, IP12 1AP, UK
www.kudosbooks.com
Kudos is a Trademark of Top That! Publishing plc

Contents

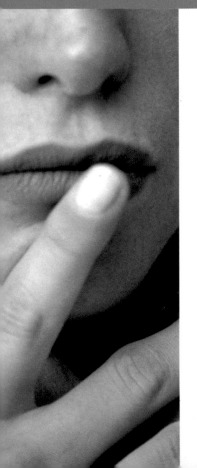

Nails Through the Ages 3

Beautiful Nails 4

The Basics 10

Shaping 12

Buffing 14

Polish 16

Maintaining
your Manicure 20

Not so Natural 24

Creating your
own Designs 28

Pedicure and
Feet Treats 42

Other Nail Treats 44

Nail Care 46

Conclusion 48

INTRODUCTION

Our love of nails has a long history. During the Chinese Ming Dynasty (1368–1644), aristocratic ladies chose to grow their nails up to ten inches long. Ever since, ladies have enjoyed nails as a fashion accessory. However, nails do have a practical purpose, and everybody should, at the very least, choose to maintain healthy nails. This kit will show you how to achieve nails to be proud of. First, though, let's take a sweeping look at our love affair with nails since the nineteenth century.

NAILS THROUGH THE AGES

1800S

Elegant, short, almond shaped nails were the fashion. A European doctor named Sitts developed the orangewood stick in 1830 – slightly more gentle than the acid and scissors previously used to shape nails. Salons in the US offered nailcare to women from all walks of life.

1900-1919

A nail varnish was invented, but it rubbed off in a day. Metal scissors allowed women to cut their nails. Cutex® made a manicure set, consisting of polish, cuticle remover, whitener and an orangewood stick.

1920-1939

Nail polish entered the market, using car paint as inspiration. The first colour was a mid-red and was only applied to the centre of the nail. The 'moon manicure' was the latest craze – ladies cut their cuticles, then applied polish to the nail but not the white 'crescent' on the nail plate.

1940-1959

Long, red talons were in vogue. Clear polish was introduced. By 1950, the fashion for pointed nails gave way to a more practical oval. Precision instruments designed especially for the manicure hit the market.

1960-1979

A riot of nail colours was available but pale colours were the popular option of the early sixties. The seventies heralded the era of synthetic nails. In 1978, the US manufacturer Orly® introduced the first branded French manicure 'kit'.

1980-1999

Nail products such as hardener and strengthener hit the shops. Artificial nails became very popular when the introduction of new materials such as Teflon™-induced acrylic made for a smooth, professional finish. Nail art took off: rhinestones, piercings and complex polish designs were available in nail bars.

3

Beautiful Nails

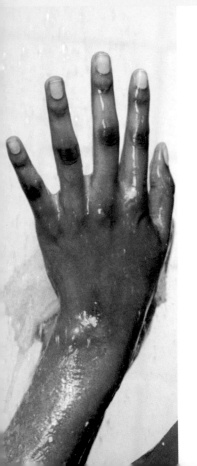

This kit will show you how to make the most of your nails and help to transform them into something special. Nails are surprisingly practical structures with two main purposes. The fingernail itself is made from a tough substance called keratin which, as well as acting as a protective sheet, has an important sensory function. The pressure our nails are put under sends information about objects to the fingers and allows us to judge the hardness of a marble table-top, or the softness of cotton wool, for example.

NAIL STRUCTURE

NAIL BED

The keratin sheet is just the surface. Beneath the sheet itself lies the nail bed, which is known as the sterile matrix. It contains the nerve endings and blood vessels.

Nail Root

The root of the fingernail is known as the germinal matrix. This part lies behind the nail and extends several millimetres into the finger. If you look at the half-moon shape at the base of the nail plate, which is called the lunula, you'll see the edge of the germinal matrix.

Nail Plate

The nail plate itself looks pink due to the blood vessels lying underneath it. As the nail grows from the root, it joins itself to a material from the nail bed that makes the nail plate thicker.

Cuticle

Also known as the eponychium, this thin strip at the base of the nail fuses the nail bed to the nail plate, and works as a waterproof barrier against infection.

Perionychium

This is the skin at the side of the nail plate. It is an area that can easily be damaged and is often the site of unattractive hangnails and infection.

plate

lunula

nail bed

cuticle (eponychium)

perionychium

GROWTH

Nails never stop growing, but the rate of growth slows as we grow older. Whatever age we are, poor circulation is also a factor in slow nail growth. If you were to lose an entire nail, it would take twelve to eighteen months to grow back completely.

HEALTHY NAILS

Our nails undergo varying degrees of wear and tear. They are often neglected and it's important to examine your nails under a good light to diagnose any problems that are directly related to your lifestyle. Here are a few of the most common nail complaints:

WHITE SPOTS

Look at the nail plate. Are there white spots dotting the pink surface? There are two main theories as to why these spots appear. Firstly, the day-to-day wear and tear on the hands means that bumps to the nail bed cause bruises which eventually appear as flecks. The other school of thought argues that a lack of zinc in the diet may be a factor – so start eating more spinach! In any case, you will have to wait for the entire nail plate to grow out before they disappear.

RIDGES

The medical name for this condition is onychorrhexis. Ridges are common in older people and there is little you can do to get rid of them. Both horizontal and 'longitudinal' (vertical) ridges may be a reflection of your diet. Ensure that you get enough vitamins and minerals. Vitamin supplements may help, and try to eat five portions of fruit and vegetables every day.

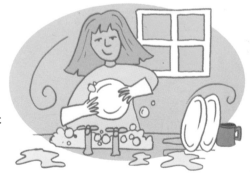

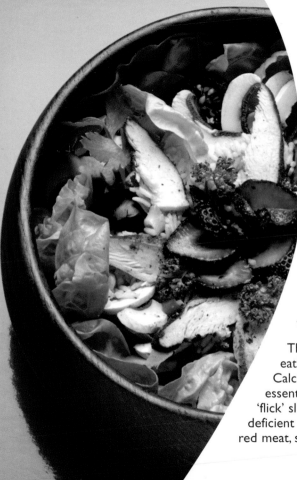

Brittle Nails

Brittle and dry nails that split easily may be due to the amount of time your hands spend in water. Try to wear rubber gloves when doing the washing up. Constant wear of synthetic nails may also cause weak spots if they are not removed very carefully. After your nails have been in contact with water for extended periods of time, for example, after swimming or bathing, massage a rich moisturiser into the nail and towards the cuticle.

Weak, Curved Ends

The old cliché that 'we are what we eat' holds particularly true with nails. Calcium for strong nails and bones is essential. If your nails do not lie flat, and 'flick' slightly at the ends, you could be deficient in iron, so again, get extra iron from red meat, spinach and watercress.

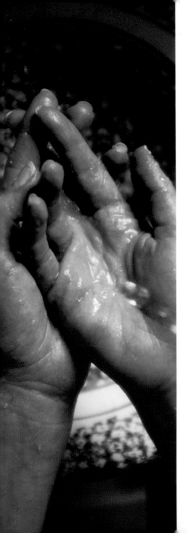

Infection

Whilst the conditions mentioned are often unsightly, they do not represent any threat to your health (although they may be symptoms of an underlying problem). However, infections of the nail should be acted upon immediately as they can lead to pain.

Anyone can get a nail infection and it is fairly common, especially in adults. The vital thing is to treat it as early as possible. Fungal infections have three main stages. Discolouring of the tip (to yellow or brown), indicates a mild infection. If the nail thickens, becomes brittle and starts to move from the nail bed, then the bacteria has been allowed to develop further. If left untreated, the nail could develop a severe fungal infection. It will become very discoloured and brittle, and in some cases, may fall off completely.

Tell-Tale Signs

• If you notice pain, for example when putting on your tights or typing at a keyboard, then the nail could be infected. The infection enters from under the tip and spreads to the nail bed. To ensure that this doesn't happen, remember the following:

• Don't trim cuticles – the removal of the waterproof layer could result in disaster as its primary purpose is to keep germs out!

• Wash your hands regularly with soap and water, and remember to dry them thoroughly afterwards with a clean towel.

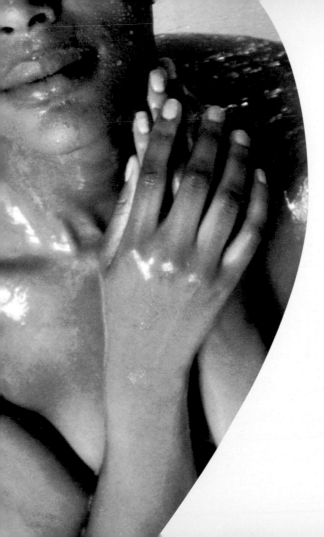

ONE MORE CLOSE LOOK...

Take a light-hearted look at what your nails reveal about your personality:

Narrow nails may indicate that you are a delicate and sensitive person. Broader nails are a sign of a frank, sensible type. 'Nail-biters' beware, – you are seen as being hypercritical!

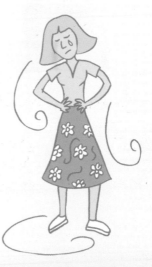

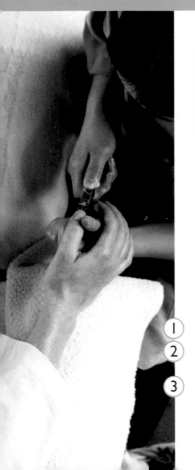

Preventing infection and achieving a basis for healthy nail growth is the vital starting point. Looking after the nail plate is the next step to giving yourself great-looking nails.

CUTICLE CARE

The thin strip of skin at the base of your nail is known as the cuticle. If you have hangnails – where the skin at the side of the nail is torn away – your cuticles may be too dry. It is very important to treat the cuticles with care. Never cut them. Simply using cuticle remover and an orange stick will do the trick. Keep your cuticles neat, clean and looking good with the following step-by-step guide.

1. Apply cuticle remover liberally to each nail in turn.

2. Hold the orange stick in a similar way to holding a pen and gently push the cuticle back.

3. Move the orange stick gently in tiny circles around the base of the nail to remove any dry skin.

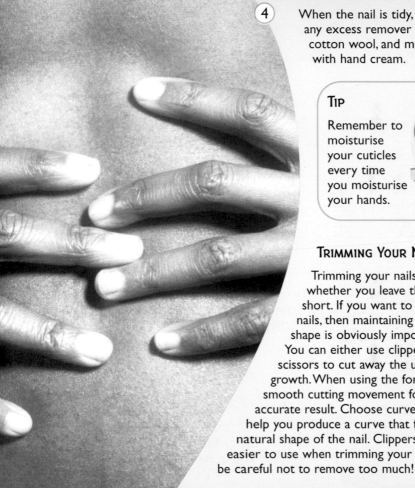

4 When the nail is tidy, wipe away any excess remover with a ball of cotton wool, and moisturise well with hand cream.

TIP

Remember to moisturise your cuticles every time you moisturise your hands.

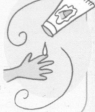

TRIMMING YOUR NAILS

Trimming your nails is vital, whether you leave them long or short. If you want to grow longer nails, then maintaining the basic shape is obviously important. You can either use clippers or scissors to cut away the unwanted growth. When using the former, use a smooth cutting movement for an accurate result. Choose curved blades to help you produce a curve that follows the natural shape of the nail. Clippers are often easier to use when trimming your toenails, but be careful not to remove too much!

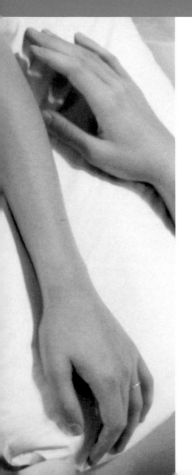

After you've established the basic length of the nail by trimming, you'll need to give it some shape. You can use a nail file for this purpose. There are both metal and synthetic emery boards on the market, although emery boards tend to be kinder to nails.

Follow the tips below to ensure that filing is a painless operation:

• File nails in one direction only.

• Replace the file frequently.

• It should take only a few light strokes of the file to get the shape you desire.

• Do not file from side to side as this goes against the direction of the nail growth and will weaken it.

• Go from one corner to the centre in one direction, and repeat on the other side. Follow the nail's natural curve.

• Leave it until the nail has grown three millimetres from the fingertip before filing, otherwise you will put undue pressure on the nail bed and this will in turn weaken the nail plate.

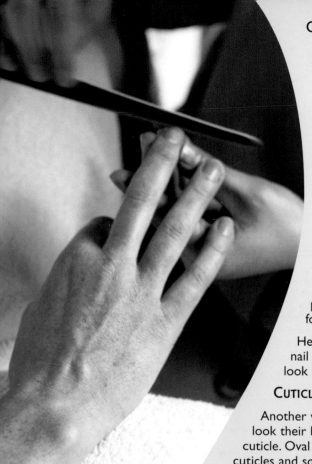

Choosing a Shape

The most important thing to remember is to follow the nail's natural curve. The shape of the tip is up to you. The key to finding a shape that suits you is to look at your hands.

Petite and fine-boned? Try 'almond' tips if you want a dramatic look, as they will lengthen and complement your fingers.

Long and slim, or short and stocky? The 'squoval' (a cross between a square and an oval) is the shape for you. Highly versatile and more practical than pointed nails, the squoval is great for a more fashionable look.

Heavy hands and wide nail bed? Try nail extensions to make your hands look more elegant.

Cuticle Clues

Another way to ensure that your nails look their best is to follow the shape of the cuticle. Oval nails complement deep, oval cuticles and squoval nails look good if your cuticles are more shallow.

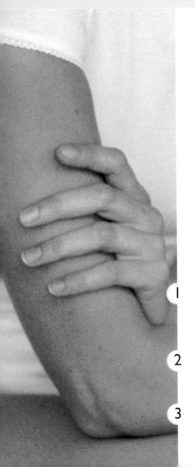

If you prefer the totally natural look, or are short of time, buffing is a great way of making your nails gleam.

There are several types of buffer available, some with only a single surface, others with three sides. Single surface buffers require the same movement with firm to light pressure. Three-sided buffers require slightly more effort, but follow these easy steps for a super shiny finish.

STEP BY STEP GUIDE TO BUFFING

1   Grip the buffer in your stronger hand and place the pink side on the nail. Slide it slowly back and forth, working from base to tip.

2   Repeat this with the white part of the buffer, using fairly light pressure, until your nails start to shine.

3   Finish with the grey side to make nails really gleam. For a natural gloss to your nails, buff them once or twice a month.

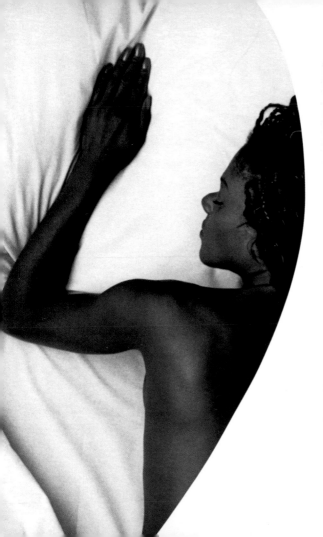

Tip

If you follow these steps to buffing, then you won't damage your nails. Although the look achieved by buffing is addictive, you should not do it more than once a week. Be gentle!

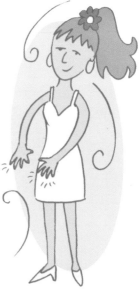

Polish

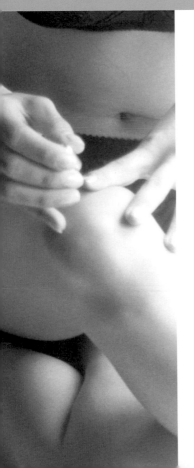

Whether you desire the classic look of a French manicure, prefer a simple touch of top coat, or want brilliant fire-engine red on your toenails as well as your fingernails, your choice of polish says something about your mood.

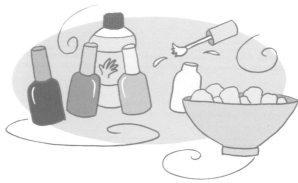

APPLYING POLISH

Different looks require various types of application, but the basic piece of equipment you'll be using is a brush. Almost every nail polish design needs to be done in three stages: base coat, colour, then top coat.

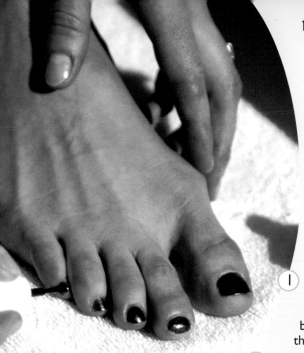

BASE COAT

The application of a primer (base coat) will prevent coloured nail varnish staining your nails. To speed up the process, find a fast-drying base coat. Apply it in a thin, even coat and allow it to dry completely.

THE COLOUR

With practice you will soon be able to paint on polish quickly and neatly.

1. Firstly, shake the bottle to ensure that the colour is evenly mixed. Dip the brush into the bottle and wipe off any excess on the neck of the bottle.

2. Apply one stroke down the centre of the nail.

3. Follow with two more strokes, one down each side, acquiring more polish from the bottle if required.

4. Leaving a tiny gap above the cuticle will give you a professional look.

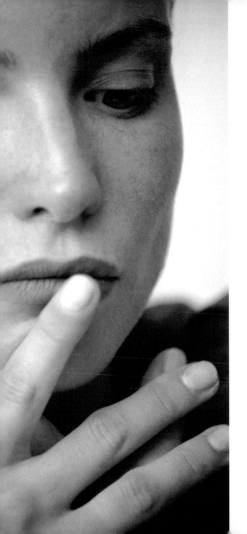

Top Coat

Again, this is vital for a really professional look and will help to maintain the 'life' of the polish. Apply a thin layer of top coat to seal and give a glossy finish.

Tips

• Be careful not to use too much polish – it is far better to apply two thin coats, rather than one thick, lumpy layer.

• Practice! Applying nail polish is a skill that needs a steady hand. Once you have mastered the art of a single colour, you'll be able to tackle more detailed designs with confidence.

• Use the entire brush, not just the tip (unless you are doing details.) If the strands are 'flattened' against the nail you will achieve thinner, smoother layers of polish.

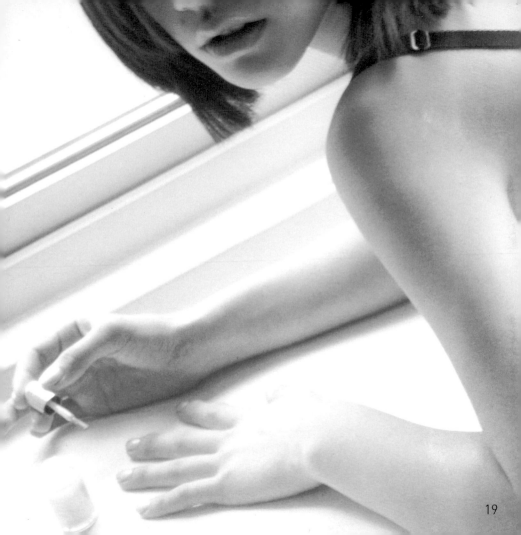

Maintaining your Manicure

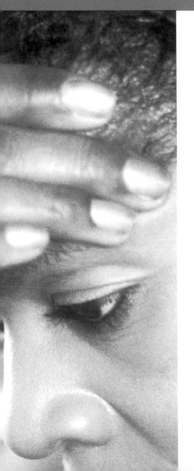

To make your manicure last as long as possible, it is important that you start with clean, dry nails. The natural oils produced by the nail itself will make the polish peel. Always use a base and a top coat to act as a foundation and sealant for the polish. Wear gloves for gardening and washing up.

REPAIRING

It is highly irritating to chip your freshly-applied nail polish. If this happens, apply another coat of polish and seal with top coat. To reduce the likelihood of this occurring, seal the polish with a layer of top coat every other day.

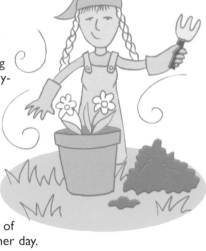

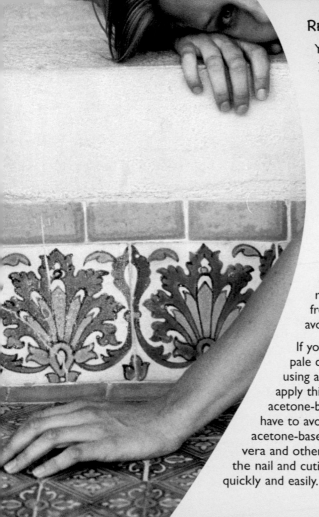

Removal

You can mend a few chips to your manicure, but nothing looks worse than layers of highly chipped polish. There are several products you can use for removing old polish.

The first is acetone-based remover. This has lost its initial popularity because it dries cuticles and weakens nails. Used carefully, however, it takes some beating for removing layers of highly coloured polish. Place some cotton wool on the end of an orange stick, dip it into the remover and swab the polish from the nail ensuring that you avoid your cuticles.

If your manicure only consists of a pale colour or a top coat, it is worth using acetone-free remover. You can apply this in the same way as an acetone-based remover but you don't have to avoid the cuticle area. The latest acetone-based removers, containing aloe vera and other moisturisers, are gentler on the nail and cuticles while still removing polish quickly and easily.

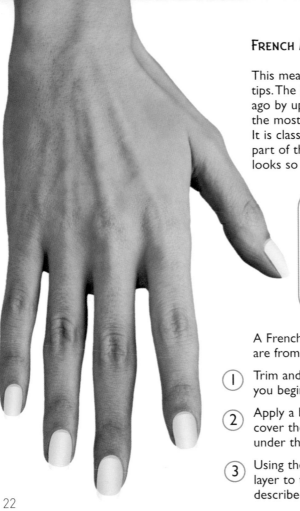

FRENCH MANICURE

This means pink nails with bright-white tips. The look was pioneered 70 years ago by upper class French ladies, and is the most requested look at salons today. It is classic, polished, yet natural. Perhaps part of the enduring appeal is that it looks so professional.

YOU WILL NEED

- Base coat
- Pink, white and clear polish
- Nail guards (available from chemists and some supermarkets)

A French manicure looks best on nails that are from six to twenty millimetres in length.

1. Trim and file your nails into shape before you begin.

2. Apply a base coat. Use only a thin layer, and cover the entire nail and brush a little under the tip. Leave to dry thoroughly.

3. Using the pink polish provided, apply a thin layer to the entire nail in three strokes as described on page 17.

(4) Find the white polish from the kit. Dip the brush into the bottle, wipe off the excess, and paint the nail tip, by stroking from the outside corner of each side towards the centre. Alternatively, apply a stick-on nail guard below the tip of the nail. Paint the tip white, stroking from the top of the guide and away from the nail. Be very careful to ensure that no polish goes below the nail guard.

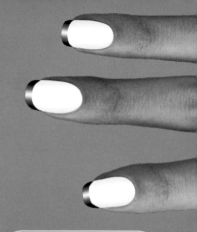

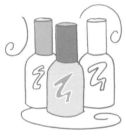

(5) Let the tips dry thoroughly. Remove the guards, if used, by carefully peeling them from one side of the nail to the other.

(6) Apply a layer of top coat over the entire nail, including the tips. Let this dry! This will seal in the layers of polish and give a great, glossy finish.

VARIATIONS

• In recent years there have been many twists on the classic French manicure. Why not try these combinations for a subtle change?

• Reverse French – black tips, white nails.

• American – beige or neutral nails with white tips.

• Modern – try luminous tips and white nails!

23

Not so Natural

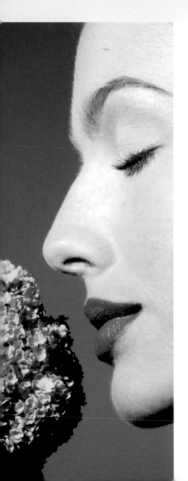

If you have a yearning for long, well-shaped nails or want a quick fix for a fabulous night out, artificial nails may be for you.

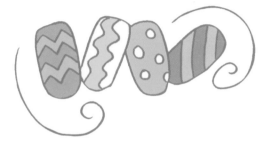

There are two main ways of applying artificial nails. The first involves putting a piece of fibreglass, acrylic or gel over the nail, which is then 'sculpted' into the shape and to the length you want. This is known as an 'overlay'. When your natural nail grows underneath, the manicurist will re-touch the area at the base of your nail with polish and file down the artificial tip. This is known as a 'fill' and needs re-touching every two to three weeks. Fibreglass nails are very thin and give perhaps the most natural look. Acrylic nails are thicker and there may be a slight 'ridge' where the 'overlay' joins the base of the nail plate. Eventually, your natural nail should be the same length as the overlay.

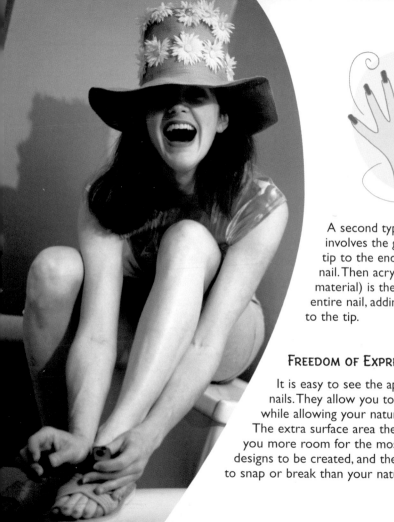

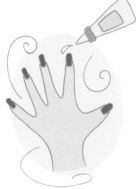

A second type of application involves the gluing of a plastic tip to the end of your natural nail. Then acrylic (or similar material) is then laid over the entire nail, adding extra strength to the tip.

FREEDOM OF EXPRESSION

It is easy to see the appeal of artificial nails. They allow you to enjoy long talons while allowing your natural nails to grow. The extra surface area they provide gives you more room for the most intricate of designs to be created, and they are less likely to snap or break than your natural nails.

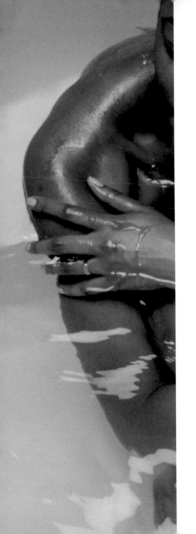

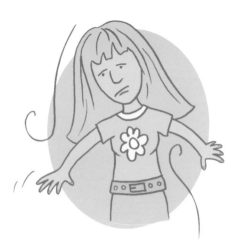

High Maintenance

To keep artificial nails looking good you must visit a manicurist or 'nail bar' every two to three weeks, and you must ensure that you look after them, in the meantime.

Applying undue pressure on your artificial nails may cause the overlays to 'lift' from the natural nail. Once the space between the nail bed and nail plate is no longer airtight, bacteria can enter freely and turn your natural nail a greenish colour. If this happens, you should go straight to a professional to have the overlays removed. Never try to remove them yourself as you will cause damage to your natural nails by creating weak spots.

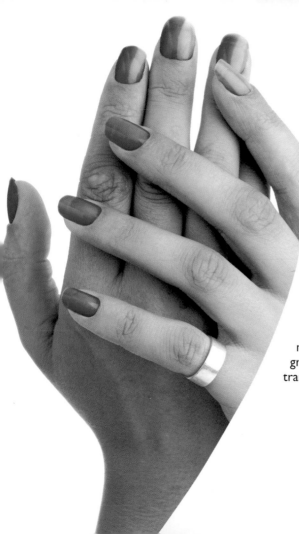

QUICK TIPS

If the idea of regular trips to the beauty salon puts you off, then there's no reason why you can't do it yourself at home. There are a variety of artificial nails on the market and many claim to strengthen your own nails. You can buy good quality kits from drugstores or beauty salons, and they're reasonably priced. Always make sure that all products have been dermatologist and salon tested.

Artificial nails applied at home might not last as long, but they are great for a quick and easy transformation.

Creating your own Designs

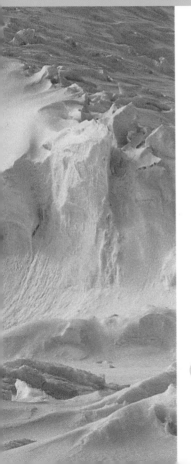

You don't have to go to the professionals to achieve stunning nails. Here are some designs you may wish to try, on both natural and synthetic nails.

SNOW LEOPARD

YOU WILL NEED:

- Base coat
- White polish
- Black polish
- Silver polish
- Clear polish
- A cocktail stick

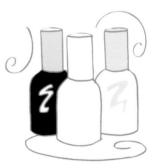

1. Apply a clear polish base coat to all nails.

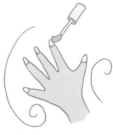

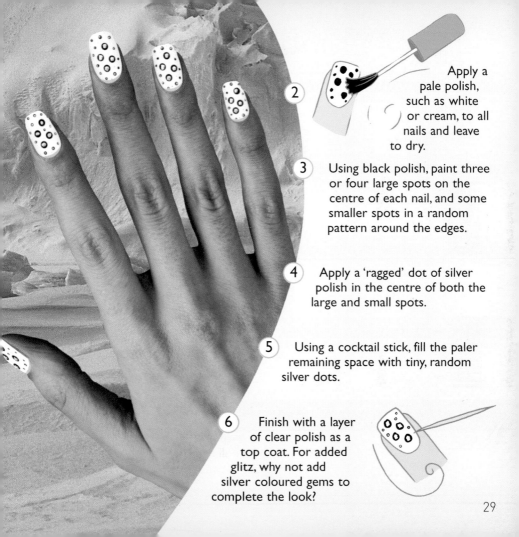

2 Apply a pale polish, such as white or cream, to all nails and leave to dry.

3 Using black polish, paint three or four large spots on the centre of each nail, and some smaller spots in a random pattern around the edges.

4 Apply a 'ragged' dot of silver polish in the centre of both the large and small spots.

5 Using a cocktail stick, fill the paler remaining space with tiny, random silver dots.

6 Finish with a layer of clear polish as a top coat. For added glitz, why not add silver coloured gems to complete the look?

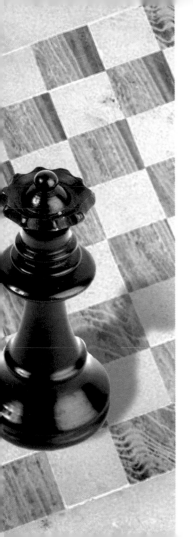

CHESSBOARD

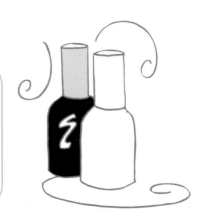

YOU WILL NEED:
- Base coat
- Black polish
- White polish
- A cocktail stick
- Clear polish

(1) Apply a clear polish base coat to all nails.

(2) Apply a bright, white polish to all nails and leave to dry.

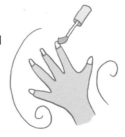

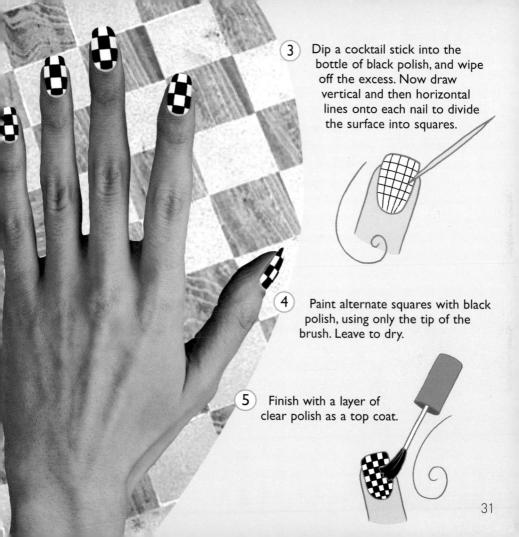

3 Dip a cocktail stick into the bottle of black polish, and wipe off the excess. Now draw vertical and then horizontal lines onto each nail to divide the surface into squares.

4 Paint alternate squares with black polish, using only the tip of the brush. Leave to dry.

5 Finish with a layer of clear polish as a top coat.

31

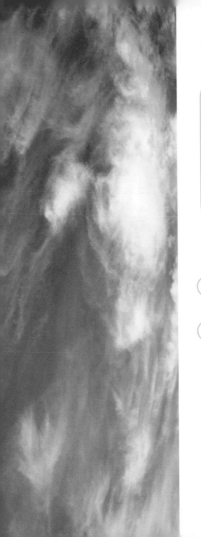

DREAMY SKY

YOU WILL NEED:

- Blue polish
- White polish
- Cocktail stick
- Pale glittery polish
- Clear polish

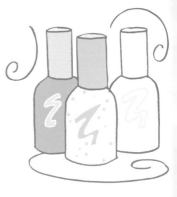

(1) Apply clear polish as a base coat to all nails.

(2) Apply a medium blue polish to all nails and leave to dry.

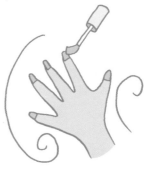

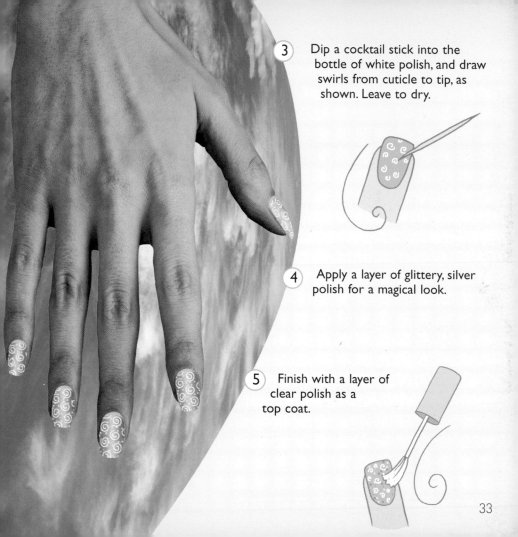

3 Dip a cocktail stick into the bottle of white polish, and draw swirls from cuticle to tip, as shown. Leave to dry.

4 Apply a layer of glittery, silver polish for a magical look.

5 Finish with a layer of clear polish as a top coat.

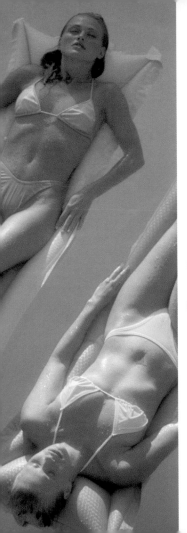

Two Halves

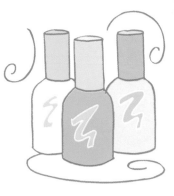

YOU WILL NEED:

- A cocktail stick
- Yellow polish
- Green polish
- Silver polish
- Clear polish

1) Apply clear polish as a base coat to all nails.

2) Dip a cocktail stick in the bottle of yellow polish, and draw a sweeping curve vertically along the length of each nail, dividing the area roughly in half, as shown.

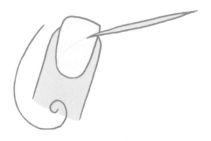

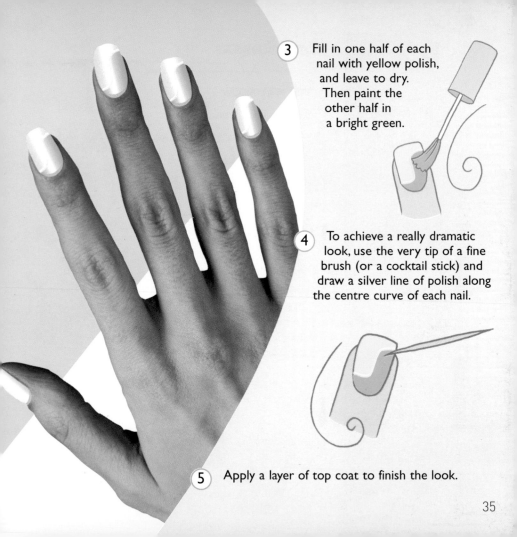

3. Fill in one half of each nail with yellow polish, and leave to dry. Then paint the other half in a bright green.

4. To achieve a really dramatic look, use the very tip of a fine brush (or a cocktail stick) and draw a silver line of polish along the centre curve of each nail.

5. Apply a layer of top coat to finish the look.

35

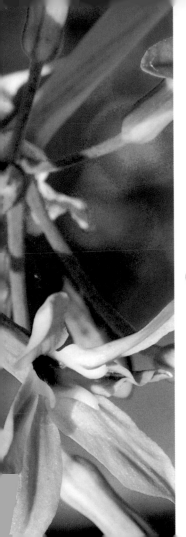

Fresh Flowers

You will need:

- White base coat
- Multicoloured glitter polish
- A cocktail stick
- Blue 3D polish (ask at your local nail salon)
- Clear polish

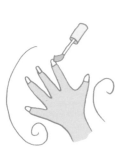

1. Apply a white or pearlescent base coat to all nails.

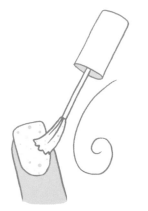

2. Apply a layer of glitter polish to all nails.

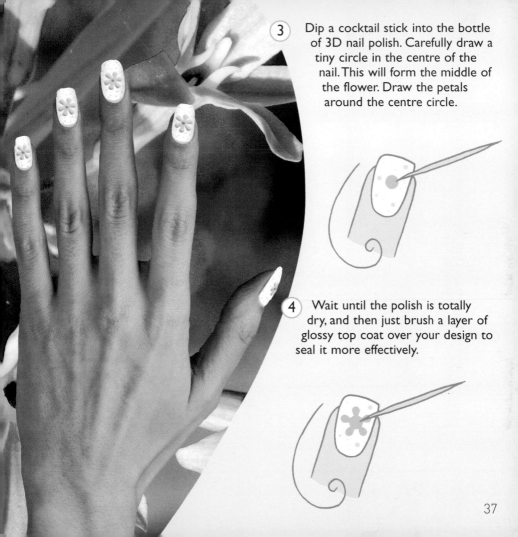

3 Dip a cocktail stick into the bottle of 3D nail polish. Carefully draw a tiny circle in the centre of the nail. This will form the middle of the flower. Draw the petals around the centre circle.

4 Wait until the polish is totally dry, and then just brush a layer of glossy top coat over your design to seal it more effectively.

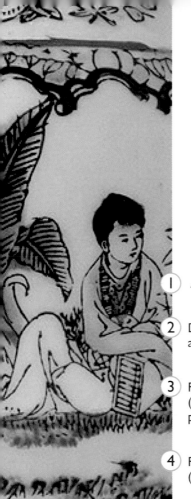

CHINESE ROSE

YOU WILL NEED:

- Gold polish
- Red polish
- A cocktail stick
- White polish

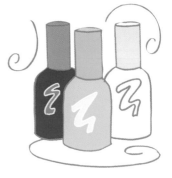

1. Apply clear polish as a base coat to all nails.

2. Draw a slanting line with gold paint, at the angle shown, on all nails.

3. Fill the area above this line (towards the cuticle) in gold polish and leave to dry.

4. Fill the area below this line (towards the tip) in red polish, and leave to dry.

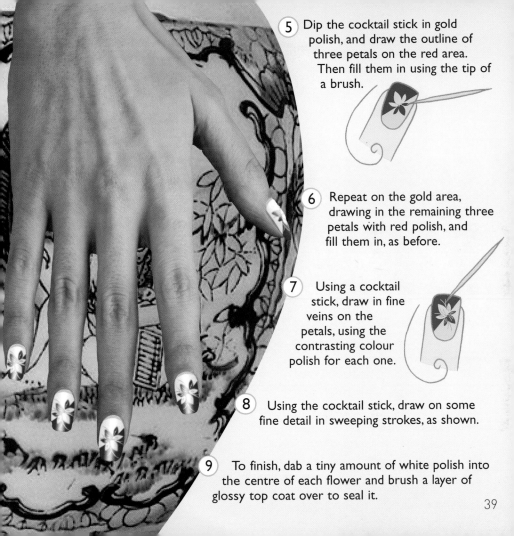

5 Dip the cocktail stick in gold polish, and draw the outline of three petals on the red area. Then fill them in using the tip of a brush.

6 Repeat on the gold area, drawing in the remaining three petals with red polish, and fill them in, as before.

7 Using a cocktail stick, draw in fine veins on the petals, using the contrasting colour polish for each one.

8 Using the cocktail stick, draw on some fine detail in sweeping strokes, as shown.

9 To finish, dab a tiny amount of white polish into the centre of each flower and brush a layer of glossy top coat over to seal it.

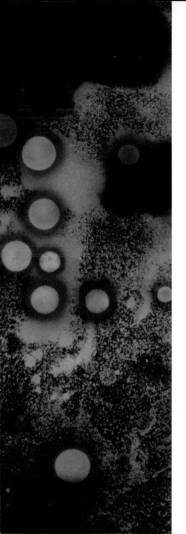

Starburst

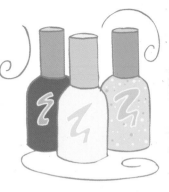

(1) Apply clear polish as a base coat to all nails.

(2) Paint each nail dark pink and leave to dry.

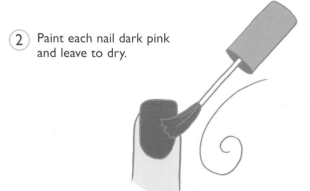

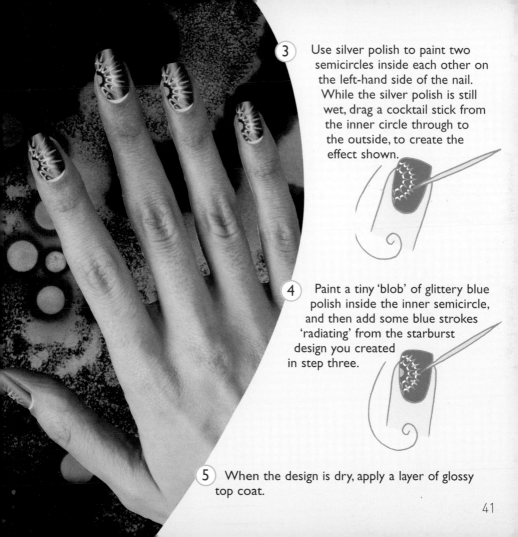

3 Use silver polish to paint two
semicircles inside each other on
the left-hand side of the nail.
While the silver polish is still
wet, drag a cocktail stick from
the inner circle through to
the outside, to create the
effect shown.

4 Paint a tiny 'blob' of glittery blue
polish inside the inner semicircle,
and then add some blue strokes
'radiating' from the starburst
design you created
in step three.

5 When the design is dry, apply a layer of glossy
top coat.

41

Pedicure and Feet Treats

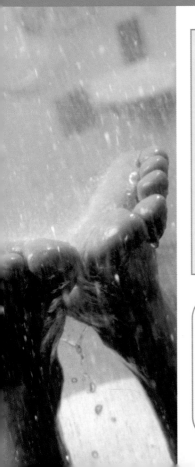

PEDICURES

Whatever the weather, our fingernails are always on show. But be wary of neglecting your other nails! Our feet spend most of their time stuffed into socks and shoes, and the onset of a hot day may be a cause for dismay when you are forced to reveal out-of-condition toenails. A pedicure every ten to fourteen days will keep your feet looking beautiful. Try this one out at home:

YOU WILL NEED:

- Orange stick (from the kit)
- A rich moisturiser
- Warm, soapy water
- A towel
- Nail scissors or clippers
- An emery board
- A pumice stone
- Toe separator

Tip

It is important to apply a layer of base coat to your toenails, as they, too, can also be stained by nail polish. The application of a top coat will leave an attractive finish.

1. If you have a foot spa, soak your feet in lots of warm, bubbly water. If not, fill a bowl with warm, soapy water and immerse your feet until they are squeaky clean.

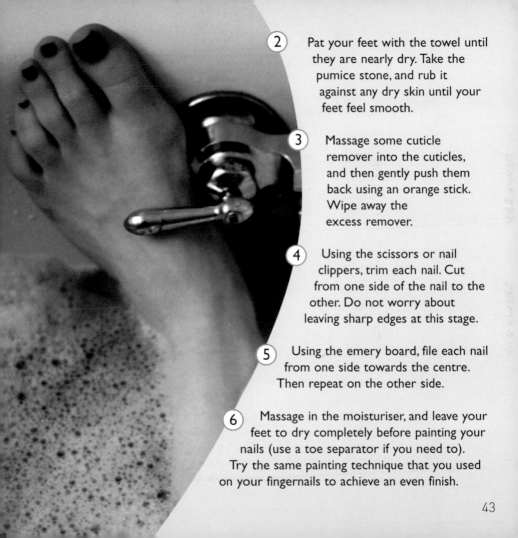

2 Pat your feet with the towel until they are nearly dry. Take the pumice stone, and rub it against any dry skin until your feet feel smooth.

3 Massage some cuticle remover into the cuticles, and then gently push them back using an orange stick. Wipe away the excess remover.

4 Using the scissors or nail clippers, trim each nail. Cut from one side of the nail to the other. Do not worry about leaving sharp edges at this stage.

5 Using the emery board, file each nail from one side towards the centre. Then repeat on the other side.

6 Massage in the moisturiser, and leave your feet to dry completely before painting your nails (use a toe separator if you need to). Try the same painting technique that you used on your fingernails to achieve an even finish.

43

Other Nail Treats

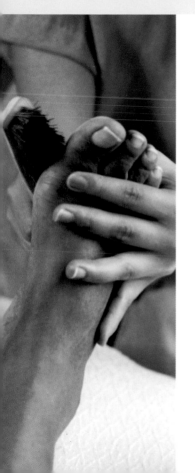

Exfoliation

When you're in the bath, brush the hard skin areas of your feet with a bristle brush to remove any rough skin. Massage some petroleum jelly into the ball and heel of each foot, then pop on a pair of socks and leave them on overnight.

Tired Soles

If you have tired feet, rub the soles with vinegar or lemon juice for a cooling, healing effect. Alternatively, stir one teaspoon of vinegar into a carton of natural yoghurt, and rub over your feet. And why not give yourself a foot massage? Rest your foot on a supportive cushion and use small, kneading movements to stimulate the multitude of nerve endings located in the soles of the feet.

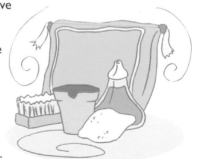

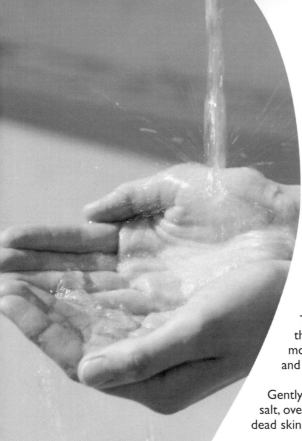

BEAUTIFUL HANDS

The sun, age and hormones may wreak havoc on your skin and make your hands look dry and papery, and ultimately, make you look older than you are. The same tips for keeping your nails looking good can be applied to your hands.

Avoid washing, or showering, in very hot or cold water as your skin will become dry and your nails brittle as they swell or shrink.

Put on some hand cream before pulling on a pair of rubber gloves. The heat that builds up inside the rubber will act as an intensive moisurising treatment for your nails and skin.

Gently rub a facial scrub, or some sea salt, over your hands to exfoliate away dead skin and keep them smooth.

Don't neglect your hands when you are applying sunscreen.

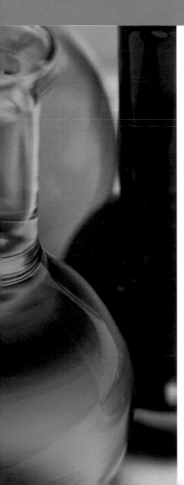

PRODUCTS

Diet and basic grooming remain the key to maintaining great nails. However, some of us are predisposed to nails that split, or are prone to weak spots and hangnails, and there are a range of products you can try that will give your nails a little extra help.

CUTICLE REPAIR

If your cuticles are dry, or you suffer from painful, raw hangnails, a regular night-time treatment may be beneficial. Look out for products that contain vitamins A, B-complex, D, E and Panthenol, as this combination of ingredients is soothing on the damaged areas.

CUTICLE OIL

Similar to products that aim to heal cuticles, these are made from a blend of healing essences which nourish these delicate areas and fight bacterial infection.

GROWTH STIMULATOR

There is little proof that applying a chemical product to the nail itself makes your nails grow faster. The best thing you can do is to keep your cuticles healthy as this will promote growth from within.

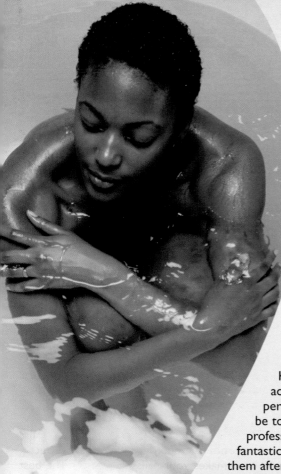

STRONGER NAILS

There are some paint-on applications that will make your nail plate stronger. The addition of a substance called Teflon™ in the fluid hardens the nail and makes it less likely to shatter and split. Applying a powder to the tip, which is removed by buffing should also make this area tougher.

ESSENTIAL OILS

If you prefer to use products with a natural base, consider essential oils. Mixing a small amount of oil with your hand or nail moisturiser will give an extra softening effect.

BITING

There is a wide range of foul-tasting, anti-biting products available. However, some nail-biters become accustomed to the bitter taste and will persist. One of the best solutions might be to apply some synthetic nails, or have a professional manicure. Your nails will look fantastic, and you may feel guilty if you bite them after spending time and money having them 'done'.

Conclusion

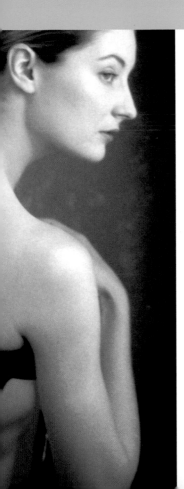

HOW DO YOU FEEL NOW?

Most people ignore their nails. Perhaps you feel a bit self-conscious devoting so much time to your hands and feet. But take a look at your nails, they look better and they feel better. There's nothing wrong with pampering yourself from time to time and there's certainly nothing wrong with having healthy nails. With healthy, good-looking nails you will feel an extra boost of confidence when meeting people; so be proud of your nails.

Perhaps the nail designs in this book will inspire you to create your own fabulous looks. Are you eager to try out your designs on your friends? Life is about having the confidence to have fun. After all, if you are going to enjoy yourself you might as well look good too!